Acquire High Energy Levels

Unleash your full potential, think clearly, gain lean muscle and lose weight

By

Lalita Chaudhari

www.lalitachaudhari.com

Website: www.lalitachaudhari.com

emailid:palmyra@lalitachaudhari.com

Dedication

This book is dedicated to my parents, Mr. P.D. Achyut and Mrs. Indira Achyut, for their unconditional love, support, and encouragement.

Disclaimer

This book is for educational purposes only. The author does not claim any medical benefits nor does she advocate any specific practice to be followed.

CONTENTS

Introduction 6

Part 1 - Affirmations 10

Part 2 - Visualization 15

Part 3- Breathwork 21

Part 4- Get Rid of Toxicity from Mind and Body 26

Part 5- Food and Fasting 33

Conclusion 39

May I ask you a favor? 40

Full Book Summary 41

About the author 45

References 46

Introduction

If you have picked up this book, chances are that you are **low on energy.** and you will find the solution to your challenge here. Whatever our age, or cultural background, life demands a level of activity from us. Our bodies are designed to heal us. This healing helps us to maximize health and happiness. We all know the importance of **physical activity** for all age groups. We shall look at five major practices to be followed that are most conducive to a favourable outcome in terms of **high energy levels.**

Now lets us look at why it is important to have **good energy levels**.

"Your days are numbered. Use them to throw open the windows of your soul to the sun. If you do not, the sun will soon set, and you with it.

Marcus Aurelius, The Emperor's Handbook

Energy is life. We must have lots of **energy** so that we can use it to serve humanity. Your biological age is determined not by the years but by the state of your body's structure and functions1.

"All that counts in life is the intention."

Andrea Bocelli

So, let's set an **intention** to have high energy levels consistently.

You may **reinforce** your intention further by having a **goal card** with the intention written. Once you have written your goal, your brain and subconscious mind get a clear message about your goal. Remember to look at the card several times a day. It is advisable to have a date by which you want to achieve this goal.

As you read **your goal aloud,** the subconscious signals become stronger. When you match these with appropriate affirmations and visuals, your **confidence** rises. Your **belief** will soar if you do this consistently.

Introduction

Key Takeaways

1) All of us can heal our bodies and thus have **high energy levels**. This book tells you how to have high energy levels.

2) It is important to have good energy levels because to do anything, you need energy.

3) In order to begin the process of achieving optimum health, (and hence optimum energy levels) set an intention. This gives the universe a **clear message** and it becomes easy for the universe to give you what you want.

4) Finally, have a **goal card** with the goal written clearly with a date for achieving the goal written on the card.

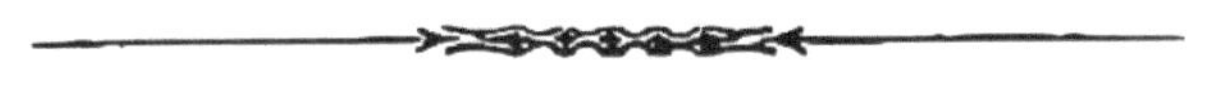

PART 1 - AFFIRMATIONS

Part 1 - Affirmations

Affirmations are real-life situations that we desire. We affirm these desires by repeating them aloud many times during the day. Affirmations **bridge the gap** between what we have and what we want. After scripting an affirmation, **say it aloud** in front of a mirror for the best results. You may also maintain a diary and write affirmations daily. Since we are affirming ourselves, these are also called self-affirmations.

Why do affirmations work?

First, we repeatedly imprint our minds with affirmations by repeating aloud or by writing. This gives a **clear message** to the brain about what we want. Soon the brain accepts this as reality by releasing the brakes.

Secondly, repetition also sends a message to the **subconscious mind**. Thus our subconscious mind knows our **vision**. Since it knows how to get there, it takes us in the right direction. If we stay in a receptive mode, we will be guided to follow the right path. Once we are on this path, we will be guided to take the right actions toward our goal achievement.

How to be in receptive mode?

Just do less left brain activity and more right brain activity. Your only job is to be easy, to be **satisfied** with where you are in your life; most important to be happy, and joyful. **Meditate** at least once a day and take a **walk in nature.**

Some affirmations that you could use -

1. I let go of all that I no longer need. My body is healing quickly and easily.

2. I have abundant energy and a strong immune system.

3. I have put my body in the hands of Mother Nature. 2

4. I am energetic, enthusiastic, and lively.

5. My score on the wellness scale is high.

What makes affirmations work?

1) In this section, we look at research done by scholars, as well as, practical applications of affirmations by world-famous life coaches.

Everyone has a basic need to maintain the **integrity of the self**. This encompasses a universal sense of personal adequacy. When this sense is threatened, stress and **feeling of inadequacy** set in. Self-affirmations can be used as interventions. Affirmations reduce stress because they bring about a more expansive view of self and resources. When affirmations are spoken or written daily, the implications of a threat to personal integrity are weakened.

"Timely affirmations have been shown to improve education, health and relationship outcomes with benefits that sometimes persist for months and years."3

2) Affirmations create an illusion of positive thinking, thereby rewiring the brain. They keep our senses **focused** on what we want. This contributes tremendously to creating our futures. 4

3) Science behind positive affirmations - Once you start repeating affirmations to yourself, the first change you may notice is a **shift in the mindset.** With a more positive attitude, you may witness a change in your habits. The actions you take to achieve your goals may seem like a **natural fit** in your life.5

4) Life Coach Tony Robbins has a system of incantations. These are affirmations that are practiced with **physiology and feelings**. This anchors them firmly in the mind.

"Everything great that has happened to humanity has begun as a single thought in someone's mind."

Yiannis Chryssomallis

Music producer, composer, and pianist

Part 1 -Affirmations

Key Takeaways

1) Affirmations are real-life situations that we **repeatedly** say aloud two or three times a day. They bridge the gap between what is and what we desire.

2) Timely affirmations have been shown to **improve education,** health, and relationship outcomes with benefits that sometimes persist for months and years.

3) When affirmations are practiced with correct physiology and emotions, they get **firmly anchored** in the mind.

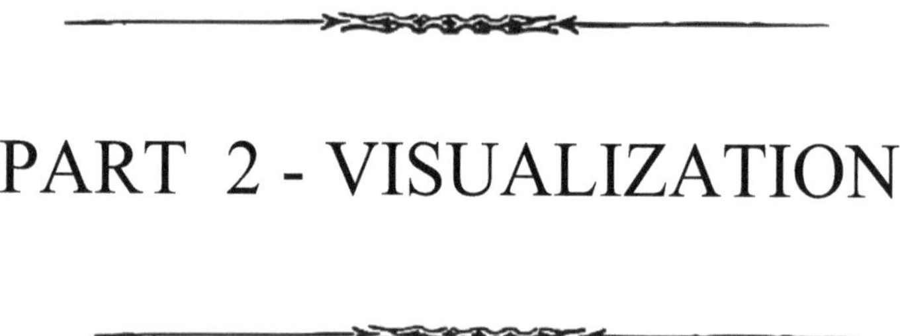

PART 2 - VISUALIZATION

Part 2 - Visualization

God has given us a wonderful ability to **think in pictures.** This is visualization. We all have dreams, things we want, places we want to visit, and so on. All these are future events, but feeling, and experiencing these as real at this moment brings us closer to achieving them. By doing this **we train our senses** about the sensations we shall be experiencing then now itself.

Thus visualization forms a big part of goal achievement. It **bridges the gap** between what is wanted and now, just like affirmations. Remember to visualize in a positive environment with lots of fun, happiness, and cheerfulness. Your subconscious mind gets activated then. It then brings incidents and thoughts into your life that take you towards your goal of having high energy.

"Make sure you visualize what you really want, not what someone else wants for you."

Jerry Gillies

Have a **goal card** with your goal written on it. You can use the one made for affirmations. This goal should have a date by which you plan to achieve it. Look at this, read it aloud, and visualize it three times a day. As you read, **visualize** how others will react, and how you will feel, and then stay with that feeling throughout the day.

Visualize how you will feel when you have lots of energy. Visualize what you will do with all the energetic new you. Now it is time to start writing some **concrete goals** in the area of finances, relationships, and contribution. Do this consistently, you will realize that your desires have an element of **certainty.** You know you will feel better and better. You are attracted to activities and humans that will help you to achieve your goals.

Let us see how this is so. Our brain has a network of nerves called the **Reticular Activating System (RAS)**6. RAS helps to focus on the important stuff. It filters the world through the parameters you give it. Our **beliefs** further shape our actions. Thus RAS helps us to remember the specific things that can help us meet the goals that we have set for ourselves. **Meditation** taps into the power of RAS. This can bring further clarity and focus.

"You visualize making a game-changing play, that's what you are here for."

Aaron Donald

Start thinking about what you want, then **reinforce** the same with visualization. Then let this drive your conscious behavior. All along know that your Reticular Activating System is working for you. Soon, your subconscious mind will get a **clearer message** and will further guide you towards achieving your goal of having high energy. Thus, **train** your mind, and your body and create the **grandest vision** you can.

Do this in a fun-filled environment, with lots of **cheerfulness**. This will take the stress away. This is important. Stress can be a fun spoiler. It affects the **immune system**. It causes inflammation in the body. Both scenarios can lead to disease (**lowering of energy**). Bad memories can play havoc too. Just change your perception of the past event. Look for what you learned and relive the memory with the changed perception. This will **heal** the subconscious mind, and when the subconscious mind heals it allows the nervous system to **relax.**

" If you do what you love, it is the best way to relax."

Christian Louboutin

A relaxed state of mind is where we want to be if not always, most of the time. Be kind to yourself. Use your **imagination** along with visualization mindfully. The visual mapping part of the brain is bigger than the other areas. **Mindfulness** is how we pay attention to ourselves; how we love ourselves. We carry ourselves not only in our minds but all over our bodies, both (mind and body) are resilient and heal themselves. Use visualization to the fullest. The bottom line is to close your eyes, sit still, and visualize what you want along with the emotions you will experience then.

Consistent practice will habituate your body and mind and soon it will **become reality.** Involve all your senses, and **sense of smell** (what will you smell, the aromas, the whiffs, the sweetness, inhalations, fragrance, incense, etc). Imagine what others will say, or what you will say to yourself. What will you perceive, foresee, notice, or observe? What will you eat, or savor? This will bring you **closer to your goal,** which seemed impossible - In other words, you will be making the impossible possible. The biggest intangible effect will be that your belief will become stronger. You will be operating comfortably outside your comfort zone now, because your **belief** has become stronger. This is crucial.

I would like to present a unique way in which visualization was used to help cancer patients. Dr. Simonton, Medical Director of the Cancer Counselling and Research Center, and the team in Fort Worth used **relaxation and visualization** techniques along with radiation therapy.

There were three basic things they asked patients to do. They asked their patients to visualize their disease, visualize their treatment, and to visualize the body's immune mechanism. The patients were asked to picture what they wanted to come about before they believed it would come about. It seemed to be important to picture it that way.7 We can use this example and apply it to your goal of having high energy levels!

Part 2- Visualization

Key Takeaways

1) God has given us the wonderful ability to think in pictures.

2) A picture is worth a thousand words, hence visualization is **powerful.**

3) Visualization works very well when affirmations have been practiced **consistently.** This is similar to a mind that has been primed.

4) Remember to be happy and playful. Visualization will not only seem to be fun then, but it will also bring in results **faster.**

5) The **consistent** practice of visualization has helped cancer patients find relief.

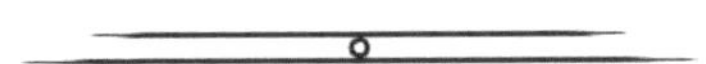

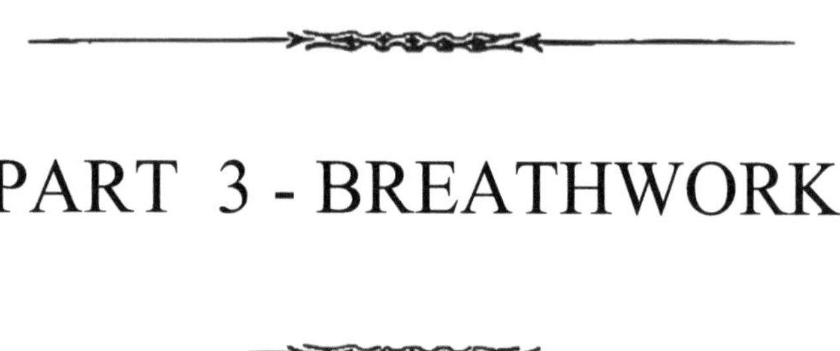

PART 3 - BREATHWORK

Part 3- Breathwork

In life, nothing and nobody will stay with you forever, except your **breath**, so, acknowledge it, honor it, and be grateful.

Let us look at this phenomenon that we take for granted. **Two** important parameters when it comes to breathing, as far as humans are concerned are -

1)   You should be breathing **5-6 breaths per minute.**

2)   If you cannot hold your breath for **more than 60seconds**, you are in the category of sick or very sick depending on the score.

It is not surprising to note that so many patients with multiple or severe health challenges have **cured themselves** by following the breathing practices taught by Swami Ramdev. There are numerous videos, as testimonials for this. Remember, that breathing does not cost a cent! It is just a matter of training yourself.

So, let me share what I follow. Note this is to be practiced **daily**. The best part is you can do this even when you are traveling. Every day as soon as I wake up, (and am still in bed), I practice **Silva Meditation**. Then, I get up, freshen up, take a cold shower, drink a glass of plain water and then follow the following breathing sequence.

i) 1 round of **Wim Hoff Breathing** method,

ii) One round of **Bellow Breathing** with 500 strokes and

iii) 27 rounds of **Alternate Nostril Breathing**. I practice this using a rosary with 108 beads. Since one round has a count of 4, it works out beautifully. It has been 3 years now, I have not missed a single day. This is followed by a 15-minute **meditation** as explained by Ester Hicks.

I have noticed three important tangible benefits of following this sequence besides high energy levels.

i) My **skin** has improved drastically. I see an improvement in muscle mass.

ii) I have not visited a doctor for any ailment, even seasonal flu or allergy. I have visited a dentist.

iii) I feel ebullient, enthusiastic, and energetic.

And this does not cost a dime!

"Breathing is the greatest pleasure in life."

Giovanni Papini

Let's look at some more benefits of breath work.

1) When you breathe deeply, you feel more alert and **more in control of your thoughts**. You become, aware of your thoughts. Thus, you control your thoughts not the other way

round. Deep breathing, thus, leads to **clarity in thoughts**. Since you also become aware of the emotions you are experiencing, you have more control over situations.

2) Deep breathing and its role in **removing toxins** from the body are often underestimated. Deep breathing causes the lungs to expand. This lets the oxygen to get absorbed easily into the blood. This is a **huge step** in making the internal body environment less acidic to slightly alkaline. This is ideal for removing tissue toxicity as well as for the cells to get nourished. Thus **blood is purified**. This is ideal for optimum functioning of all bodily systems because of the enhanced blood flow. The **lymphatic system** depends entirely on breathing for stimulation.

3) The increase in oxygen levels in the blood leads to **less stress** in the body. Deep breathing improves the health of the nervous system which includes the brain, spinal cord, and nerves. This calms the mind. When breathwork is practiced consistently anxiety, depression, and mood swings, tend to go away leading to a sense of general well-being. You **do not need drugs** to experience a sense of well-being. In my opinion, this is a HUGE PAYOFF.

4) Because of the calming effect due to breathing deeply, you tend to speak less. Your mental chatter and self-talk reduce.

Both these factors contribute to you becoming a **better listener**.

5)   Needless to say, in one way or the other, breathwork contributes to high energy levels!

Part 3 - Breathwork

Key Takeaways

1) Your breath will stay with you forever, so be **grateful**.

2) Breathe **5 to 6 times per minute**, and practice holding your breath for 60 seconds. You may start with 15 seconds, then graduate to 30 seconds, 45 seconds, and **60 seconds**.

3) Follow a system of breathing patterns. Stick to it for a lifetime. Only consistent practice bears results when it comes to **breathwork**.

4) There are many benefits of breathing deeply. These include **purifying blood**, thinking clearly, and getting rid of anxiety, depression, and many ailments.

Part 4 - Get Rid of Toxicity from Mind and Body

Part 4- Get Rid of Toxicity from Mind and Body

Why is this important?

Lets us picturise all toxic thoughts as well as toxic elements from the body going out. If you **replace** the space created with good thoughts, and good elements, since everything is energy (vibration), this will mean bad energy out, good energy in. Thus, you will have **high energy levels.**

Let us divide this section into two parts- toxicity related to our **physical body** (tangible toxicity) and toxicity related to the **mind** (intangible toxicity). Removal of toxins from the body leads to improved energy and vigor.

Regular exercise for 20-30 minutes is recommended. Do this as per your capacity. It may range from walking at your pace to going to the gym, body stretching, yoga, pilates, and weight training. The point to bear in mind is to **sweat** during exercise because sweating removes toxins from the body through the skin. Remember that skin is the largest organ for the elimination of toxins from the body.

"O, Sunlight! The most precious gold to be found on Earth."

Roman Payne

Another way in which we can use the skin to our advantage is by exposing the skin to sunlight. This should be done from sunrise till 8:30 A. M., and during the last hour before sunset. This **exposure** leads to the formation of vitamin D. This vitamin is an essential cofactor for the assimilation and utilization of Calcium in the body.

"In the Sun, I feel as one".

Kurt Cobain

Calcium, besides building the bones, and teeth, helps the body repair and detoxify. Sun gazing during the times mentioned earlier has a magical effect on pituitary and pineal glands. **Sun gazing** causes the impulses from sunlight to affect the optic nerve, retina, pituitary, and pineal glands. These glands then signal the production of essential hormones. This improves the working of the endocrine system leading to an improved **immune system**.

We all are aware of the process of **elimination** in our bodies. A well-functioning elimination process removes waste from the body. The undigested food left behind putrifies and ferments. Consuming processed food leads to malfunctioning of the elimination system. A change in diet from **processed to non-**

processed food, alongwith one that is well-balanced nutritionally will be beneficial.

Another point to keep in mind is the health of the colon. Keeping it clean will go a long way to maintaining overall good health and thus high energy levels. **Colon irrigation** would be a practice that would serve well to take proper care of the colon. Make sure to take probiotics.

"The wisdom of life consists in the elimination of non-essentials."

Lin Yutang

One way to keep the energy moving in the body is to **stimulate** the points at various locations in the body by massaging them. There are various types of massages. Some massages require professional help. In case you are not able to get professional help you can do it yourself. Just use your hands. Dip your fingers in any oil (coconut or sesame oil) and apply to your body followed by a gentle massage with your fingers. This **stimulates** the flow of toxins. Drink lots of water to flush out these toxins from your body.

Keep the body hydrated. Drink **five to eight glasses** of water every day. This will prevent dehydration as well as keep the bodily fluids alkaline and moving throughout the body. The alkaline environment and oxygen are the twin pillars of good health and strong immune response.8

Our body has tremendous power to heal itself. If you cut your finger with a blade or knife, you will notice that after some time the blood stops oozing out. The cut heals after a few days. This is a perfect example of how the body heals itself. To enhance the body's healing powers, the practice of **fasting** has been followed for ages. As per your capacity, decide the period, and type of fasting. You can start with a fast wherein you eat only fruits for a day. Some people prefer to consume only water. Others practice dry fasting. The importance of fasting lies in the fact that it leads to the production of **Human Growth Hormone (HGH)** by the glands. HGH is circulated in the body and helps to repair damaged tissues, and contributes to generating new cells.

"Through prayer, fasting and studying, God will answer."

Monica Johnson

There are non-invasive therapies like **acupuncture and acupressure** that stimulate various points on various meridians in the body. This stimulation leads to an improved flow of energy in the body, thus contributing to **improved energy levels.** Acupuncture requires professional help whereas acupressure can be practiced by anyone after gaining basic knowledge of the location of points corresponding to various organs. I call it my handy therapy.

Today, it is impossible to imagine life without electr**onic devices.** However, these should be used prudently. Microwaves, ovens, hair dryers, laptops, and mobile phones should be used with caution. Two simple ways to be on the safe side would be 1) Keep these gadgets away from your cooking as well as from your sleeping area. 2) Practice **dry fasting** for 16 hrs or as per your capacity. Dry fasting heals the body from radiation exposure.

Finally, it is important to take care of the **nervous system.** To keep the nervous system functioning at optimum levels take cold showers, practice yoga, deep breathing, meditation, singing, or chanting. A good friend circle, good social relationships, being playful and having fun most of the time may seem trivial, but they contribute to staying enthusiastic as well as energetic.

Mental hygiene - Along with practicing hygiene in the physical realm you need to follow mental hygiene also. Our thoughts are also a form of energy. Each thought carries a vibration. **Low-vibration** thoughts correspond to diseases as well as low energy and vice versa. What you think, feel, and believe in will become a reality. Remove toxic thoughts, and practice forgiveness. Be kind, loving, and gentle. This will not only prevent energy drainage but also produce energy. Thus you will have more energy that you can utilize for creative pursuits as well as for serving humanity. Your speech, and the words you utter also have energy, so use words carefully.

Part 4 Get rid of toxicity from the body and mind

Key Takeaways

1) Removing toxicity from the body and mind makes way for all that is non-toxic. When this happens in the body, it leads to renewed **energy and vigor**. When this happens in the mind, you start **thinking clearly,** your creative juices start flowing, and your productivity increases.

2) Regular exercise, exposure to the sun, sun gazing, colon irrigation, massaging the body once in fifteen days, and drinking **6-8 glasses** of water per day can help in removing toxins from the body.

3) Fasting has many benefits, such as toning the digestive system, getting glowing skin, producing human growth hormone, and giving the body tissues a chance to repair. Dry fasting has the power to **nullify the damage done due to continuous exposure to electronic gadgets.**

4) Mental hygiene is important and thoughts form a big part of the mental space. Keep your thoughts happy and positive Practice kindness and be loving towards everybody.

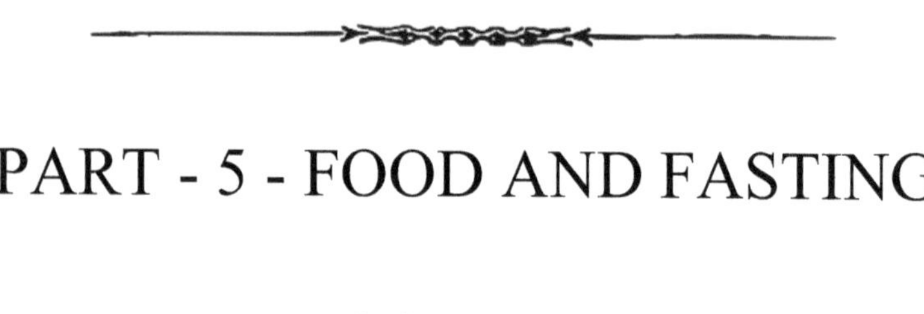

PART - 5 - FOOD AND FASTING

Part 5- Food and Fasting

Why is paying attention to food important?

We must pay attention to what we are eating, how we are eating, and when we are eating because the food we eat supplies us with energy. Hence food and everything related to is extremely important.

"Good food is the foundation of genuine happiness"

Auguste Escoffler

Along with speech, pay attention to your thoughts. This is more important when you are eating. Eating food is a divine act wherein whatever you are eating is undergoing a process to become a part of you. This is the reason to eat food with an attitude of gratitude.

Eat when the state of mind is calm. It is important to chew food well. Including a lot of greens, salads, and raw foods will improve chewing. **Thank** the farmer, Mother Nature, and everybody, whether known or unknown, for their efforts to put the food on your plate. Make sure you have washed your hands, and feet, and said a prayer of gratitude before eating. This will **improve digestion** and many challenges like allergy, constipation, indigestion, acidity will take a back seat. Do not eat when you are angry, depressed, or fearful.

"To eat is a necessity, but to eat intelligently is an art,"

Francois De LA Rochefoucals

The emotions of being courageous, **accepting,** loving, joyous, peaceful, and enlightened have high vibrations. Every other emotion is at a lower vibration. When you experience emotions with low vibration, you attract dis-ease. Easiness and **enthusiasm** are high vibrations; disease is not. So, make it a point to be in high vibration zone all the time. This is more important during eating because, as mentioned earlier, what you eat becomes a part of you. This applies to the quality of food as well. Eat high-quality food that is **alive**. Let us look at what happens once the food is ingested

Our digestive system is fantastic. A good digestive system is the foundation of good health. A well-functioning digestive system has good gut flora as its strongest pillar. **Gut flora** is also responsible for our immunity. Our immune system cannot function without constant nourishment. Stress, antibiotics, processed food, drugs, and alcohol reduce gut flora. **Fresh food**s, exposure to sunlight, and fresh air give a boost to the immune system. Good health as well as high energy levels can be achieved by living in harmony with nature. Let food be your best medicine. Even if you are eating meat and eggs, make sure they are fresh and organic. **Organic foods** are much more in tune with nature than their inorganic counterparts. Since energy is life, eat vegetables, and fruits preferably.

"There are no more important ingredients of a properly constituted diet than fruits and vegetables, for they contain vitamins of every class, recognized and unrecognized."

SIR ROBERT MCCARRISON

If your liver can process dairy, have fresh milk. Most **grains** are too **acidic** and are best consumed after soaking them and cooked very well until the grains burst open. Pay attention to what you are eating, its reaction, and its suitability. This should help you to come up with a good diet plan for yourself. No need to go to a doctor or nutritionist. You know your body the best, not the doctor or nutritionist or dietician!

"If you could build muscle, you can build a mindset."

Jay Shetty

Finally, I would like to mention the most important factor for staying energetic, **active,** and mobile even in the later part of life. We need proper muscle mass to facilitate movement. Muscle mass decreases as we age. This restricts activities such as walking or dancing and getting on or off the stairs. Hence, a word about **muscle building** is deemed important here. **Muscle retention** is the most critical element of human fitness. Let us look into the process of turning on the muscle-building mechanism. For this let us look at the right physical and nutritional **triggers**.9

The main triggers (physical as well as nutritional) of your muscle genes are:

a)   Insulin

b)   Exercise/Mechanical - Weight training

c)   Fasting

d)   Amino Acids

Let us see each in detail

a)   Insulin: Insulin turns on the muscle genes. It potentiates the most powerful muscle-building hormone - testosterone, growth hormone, and insulin-like growth factors. **Anabolism** and catabolism are two parts of the metabolic activity in the body. We need to promote anabolic activity for muscle building. When insulin activity is disturbed it disturbs the anabolic activity. It is advisable to choose foods including grains that have low glycemic index.

b)   Exercise - In gyms, we often see the trainer telling us to go one step beyond our capacity be it weights or the **repetitions** during weight lifting. This sends a message to the muscle to expand its capacity and thus grow in the process.

"The last three or four reps are what makes the muscle grow".

Arnold Schwarzenegger

c) Fasting - Fasting gives **rest** to the digestive system as mentioned earlier. It **stimulates** the human growth hormone and stabilizes insulin. This is important because growth hormone builds new muscle cells as well as brain cells. During fasting since all digestive activities are at rest, the body gets a chance to remove broken proteins, and damaged cells. This, in turn, allows the creation of new cells for repairing the damaged cells. This leads to what we call rejuvenation. This has an **anti-aging** effect. Working out while fasting causes hormones to optimize which in turn leads to **muscle gain** and **weight loss**. Remember to eat and hydrate well after exercise.

d) Amino acids - Amino acids are the building blocks of the protein molecule and hence are important. Proteins build the structure of a cell. The amino acids can be further classified as branched-chain amino acids and non-branched amino acids. The branched-chain amino acids serve as nutritional **triggers** and are found in dairy products.

When insulin and testosterone are in proper balance, we move from hunger to **satiety.** This is a very important distinction. Satiety promotes the body to be **lean, strong, and muscular**. This regimen will make us strong physically and mentally.

To reiterate, we need to

1) Eat more plant-based food and less animal-based food.

2) Foods with a low glycemic index should be preferred to keep insulin levels balanced.

3) Whole foods are preferred over processed foods.

Part - 5 - Food and Fasting

Key Takeaways

1) The food we eat supplies us with energy. So, it is important to **pay attention** to what we eat.

2) Keep your mind **calm** when you eat. Eat with an attitude of gratitude. Eat high-quality food items that are plant-based mostly. Chew your food properly. Unchewed food remains undigested. It does not contribute to body-building or to supplying energy.

3) Use your best judgment to make choices when it comes to eating. Be prudent.

4) You need to stay active whatever your age. To stay active you need good levels of energy as well as good **muscle mass**. Since muscle mass decreases as you age, be wise to look into the proper food intake as well as fasting and working out regimes.

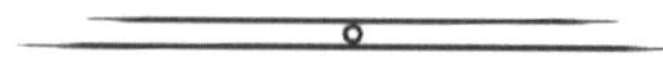

Conclusion

"Success emerges from the quality of the decisions we make and the quantity of luck we receive. We cannot control luck. But we can control the way we make choices."

-Chip Heath

Follow the five steps mentioned in this book. These are simple steps, but, following them will need discipline. It will require an indefatigable desire to succeed and a clear vision for your life. A strong desire will give you all the energy you need to succeed. Taking care of yourself is your **responsibility**!

May I ask you a favor?

I would like to thank you for taking the time to read this book. I hope you found it helpful.

May I ask for **one minute** of your time?

I would love to have you write a review for this book. This would help to improve the content. Thus, I shall be able to serve better.

Thank you for supporting my work and I look forward to reading your review.

Full Book Summary

Introduction

Key Takeaways

1) All of us can **heal our bodies** and thus have high energy levels. This book tells you how to have high energy levels.

2) This is important because to do anything, you need energy.

3)To begin the process of achieving optimum health, (and hence optimum energy levels), set an **intention**. This gives the universe a clear message and it becomes easy for the universe to give you what you want.

4) Finally, have a **goal card** with the goal written clearly with a date for achieving the goal written on the card.

Part 1 -Affirmations

Key Takeaways

1) Affirmations are real-life situations we desire that we repeatedly say aloud two or three times a day. Affirmations bridge the gap between what is and what we desire.

2) Timely affirmations have been shown to **improve** education, health, and relationship outcomes with benefits that sometimes persist for months and years.

3) When affirmations are practiced with **correct physiology** and emotions, they get firmly anchored in the mind.

Part 2- Visualization

Key Takeaways

1) God has given us the **wonderful ability** to think in pictures.

2) A picture is worth a thousand words, hence visualization is powerful.

3) Visualization works very well when affirmations have been practiced consistently. This is similar to a mind that has been primed.

4) Remember to be happy and **playful**. Visualization will not only seem to be fun then but, it will also bring in results faster.

5) The consistent practice of visualization has helped cancer patients find relief.

Part 3 - Breathwork

Key Takeaways

1) Your breath will stay with you forever, so be **grateful.**

2) Breathe **5 to 6 times per minute**, and practice holding your breath for 60 seconds. You may start with 15 seconds, then graduate to 30 seconds, 45 seconds, and **60 seconds.**

3) Follow a system of **breathing patterns**. Stick to the system for a lifetime. Only consistent practice bears results when it comes to breathwork.

4) There are many benefits of breathing deeply. These include purifying blood, **thinking clearly,** and getting rid of anxiety, depression, and many ailments.

Part 4 Get Rid of Toxicity from the Body and Mind

Key Takeaways

1) Removing toxicity from the body and mind makes way for all that is non-toxic. When this happens in the body, it leads to renewed **energy and vigor.** When this happens in the mind, you start **thinking clearly,** your creative juices start flowing, and your productivity increases.

2) Regular exercise, exposure to the sun, colon irrigation, **massaging** the body once in fifteen days, and drinking 6-8 glasses of water per day can help in removing toxins from the body.

3) Fasting has many benefits, such as **toning the digestive system,** getting glowing skin, producing human growth hormone, and giving the body tissues a chance to repair and thus heal. **Dry fasting** has the power to nullify the damage done due to continuous exposure to electronic gadgets.

4) Mental hygiene is important and thoughts form a big part of the mental space. Keep your thoughts happy and positive.

5) Practice kindness and love everybody.

Part - 5 - Food and Fasting

Key Takeaways

1) The food we eat supplies us with **energy**. So, it is important to pay attention to what we eat.

2) Keep your mind calm when you are eating. Eat with an attitude of gratitude. Eat **high-quality food** items that are plant-based mostly. Chew your food properly. Food that is not chewed properly remains undigested and does not contribute to body-building or to **supplying energy**.

3) You are your own best judge to make choices when it comes to eating. Be prudent.

4) You need to **stay active** whatever your age. To stay active you need **good levels of energy as well as good muscle mass**. Since muscle mass decreases as you age, be wise to look into the right food intake as well as fasting and working out regimes.

Taking care of yourself is **your** responsibility!

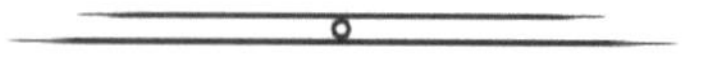

About the author

Lalita Chaudhari is a modern-day authorpreneur. A stint with an auto-immune challenge led to the path of solution finding. This has culminated in writing this book. She sincerely wishes the readers good health, prosperity, and happy life.

She earned a B.Arch from Bhopal University followed by a Masters in Urban and Regional Planning from Virginia Commonwealth University, Richmond, Virginia, USA. With a tremendous love for research as well as to share her learnings, she presents the book.

References

1 Andrew Weil, M.D., *Healthy Aging:2005* (Anchor Books), 118

2 Luke Coutinho, *The Dry Fasting Miracle,* (Pothi.com), 45

3 Geoffrey L.Cohen (Dept of Psychology, Stanford University) and David K. Sherman (Dept. of Psychological and Brain Sciences, *The Psychology of change - Self-affirmations and Social Psychological intervention,* Annual Review of Psychology, Vol 65:333-37. (Jan 2014)

4 Ayomide Obidye Mcxhem (Osun State University), *The Power of Affirmation. Creating an illusion of Positive Thinking.* Research gate.net/publication/343809400, August 2020.

5https://www.thirdspace.london/this-space/2021/02/the-science-behind-positive-affirmations/

6 If you want, you might get it. The Reticular Activating System explained by Tobias van Schneider (*blog)*

7 Jose Silva and Philip Miele, *The Silva Mind Control Method,* (Simon & Schuster, 1977), 82

8 Daniel Reed, *The Tao of Detox,* (Pocket Books), 2007, 6

9 Ori Hofmekler, *Unlock Your Muscle Gene, (North Atlantic Books, 2011),*146